WORLD WAR II Q&A

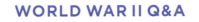

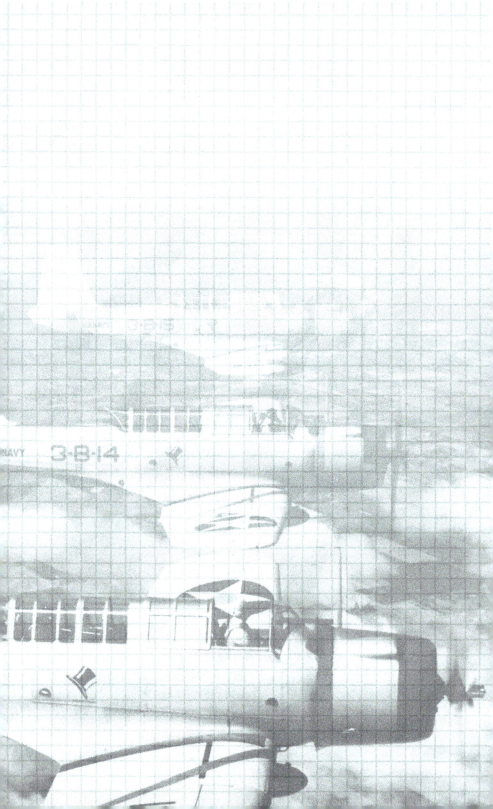

WORLD WAR II

Q&A

175+ Fascinating Facts for Kids

R. KENT RASMUSSEN

ROCKRIDGE
PRESS

**To David Balmforth: cherished friend
of my youth, US Coast Guard shipmate,
and serious student of World War II**

For general information on our other products and services or to obtain technical support, please contact our Customer Care Department within the United States at (866) 744-2665, or outside the United States at (510) 253-0500.

Rockridge Press publishes its books in a variety of electronic and print formats. Some content that appears in print may not be available in electronic books, and vice versa.

Series Designer: Diana Haas
Interior and Cover Designer: Regina Stadnik
Art Producer: Megan Baggott
Editor: Eliza Kirby
Production Editor: Jenna Dutton
Production Manager: Michael Kay

Photography & Illustration © ClassicStock/Alamy, Cover; U.S. National Archives and Records Administration, 3, 11, 20, 36, 49, 52, 61; Sueddeutsche Zeitung/Alamy, 5; Everett Historical/Shutterstock, 7, 9, 12, 40; Pictorial Press Ltd/Alamy, 16; CPA Media Pte Ltd/Alamy, 24; Alpha Historica/Alamy, 26; Lenscap Photography/Shutterstock, 27; Library of Congress, 28, 37, 43, 51, 57, 60, 64; Hum Historical/Alamy, 32; Imperial War Museum, 34; Alamy Stock Photos, 35; Michael Seleznev/Alamy, 42; Smith Archive/Alamy, 44; imageBROKER/Alamy, 45; Pictorial Press Ltd/Alamy, 47; Lt. Gaetano Faillace/US Army, 63.

Hardcover ISBN: 978-1-63878-618-4 | Paperback ISBN: 978-1-64876-774-6
eBook ISBN: 978-1-64876-383-0
R0

INTRODUCTION

World War II was the most terrible war in human history. It involved more countries, killed more people, and did more damage than any other conflict. It was a huge and complicated event, but it is easier to understand by looking at it as two mostly separate wars. One was fought mainly in East Asia and the Pacific Ocean beginning in 1937. The other was fought mostly in Europe, North Africa, and the Atlantic Ocean beginning in 1939. In late 1941, the United States entered both wars at the same time to help the United Kingdom, the Soviet Union, and other Allied nations defeat the Axis forces of Germany, Japan, and their allies.

The pages that follow answer your questions about the countries, people, weapons, and battles that made up the war and how the conflict changed the world.

Now, prepare to take a step back into one of the most momentous periods in history ...

WHAT CAUSED THE WAR?

Q Was World War II a continuation of the First World War?

A In some ways, yes. Despite the earlier war's size and horrible death toll, World War I didn't resolve every issue that had caused it. Many Germans felt they had been cheated because their country had surrendered without really losing the war. Their leader, Adolf Hitler, encouraged that belief. The Germans were willing to continue what they felt was an unfinished fight.

Q What settlement came out of World War I?

A The 1919 Treaty of Versailles came out of World War I. The terms were dictated by the major victors: Great Britain, France, Italy, and the United States. The French and British had suffered the most and wanted to punish Germany. The treaty took away Germany's colonies and some of its own territory, shrank its military forces, and required it make almost ruinous reparation payments.

TRUE OR FALSE?

US president Woodrow Wilson created the League of Nations after World War I.

MOSTLY TRUE.

Wilson was the first world leader to propose a world organization to prevent future wars, and he helped design the league. But because he could not persuade Congress to allow the United States to join, he played no role in the league's operations.

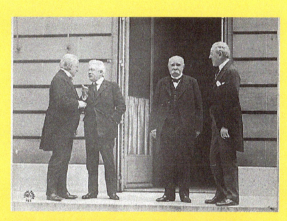

US president Woodrow Wilson (far right) with leaders of Great Britain, France, and Italy at the 1919 peace conference

Q Did the League of Nations' weakness help cause World War II?

A The league's major failure was doing nothing effective to punish Japan, Italy, and Germany's aggressive actions before the war. By 1937, Germany, Japan, and Italy had all left the league, and everyone stopped taking its peacekeeping mission seriously.

Q What was the
Weimar Republic?

A The Weimar Republic was the democratic form of government that replaced Germany's monarchy—a type of government run by a king or queen—after World War I. It ended in 1933, when Hitler became chancellor and declared Germany's "Third Reich."

Stat: During the early 1920s, Germany's currency, the mark, had one of the highest inflation rates in history. In 1919, one US dollar bought **90** German marks. By late 1923, it could buy **4.2 trillion** marks. Prices rose so fast that people had to spend their money quickly, before it lost its value.

Q What was the Munich
Beer Hall Putsch?

A The "Munich Beer Hall Putsch," which occurred in November 1923, was Hitler's first step in his takeover of Germany's government. Despite having police and army support, it failed, and Hitler went to prison. The incident made him a national figure and a **Nazi** hero.

Did You Know?

Mein Kampf ("My Struggle"), the autobiography Hitler wrote while in prison during the 1920s, made him rich. After he came to power, every Nazi family was expected to own a copy.

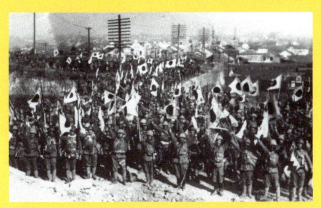

Japanese troops in Nanking, China, in 1938

Q How did the world depression help bring on the war?

A After 1929, declining national economies, widespread unemployment, bank failures, and other problems in Japan and Europe made people lose faith in democratic governments. They became more willing to accept dictators and other solutions to problems, including war. A major reason **Axis** countries went to war was to control other countries' resources.

Q What drove Japan to war?

A Japan was a rapidly modernizing island country that needed to import most of its resources. To guarantee its future power, Japan began seizing other territories in Asia during the early 1930s.

Q What was Japan's "Greater East Asia Co-Prosperity Sphere"?

A This was Japan's name for Indochina (Southeast Asia), the Philippines, Malaya, and the Dutch East Indies (now Indonesia). Japan wanted to rule these countries and use their resources.

TRUE OR FALSE?

Before World War II, Japan and the United States were on good terms.

FALSE.

Japan and the United States were allies during World War I, but things became tense in the lead-up to World War II. Japan was exercising its military power against China. The United States disapproved and cut off trade with Japan.

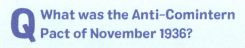

Q What was the Anti-Comintern Pact of November 1936?

A Germany and Japan agreed to oppose Soviet communism and to defend each other if the Soviet Union attacked. This agreement was called the "Anti-Comintern Pact." Italy joined the pact a year later.

Did You Know?

While future US president John F. Kennedy was studying at Harvard in the late 1930s, he wrote his senior thesis on Great Britain's failure to prepare for the coming war with Germany.

Q What was the United States doing between the wars?

A World War I left many Americans opposed to getting involved in future wars. Congress passed neutrality acts that forbade the government from taking sides in foreign conflicts. Still, President Franklin D. Roosevelt looked for ways to help the **Allies** when the war started in 1939. The great distances separating the United States from the conflicts made Americans feel safe, until Japan attacked Pearl Harbor in 1941.

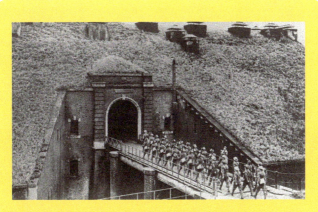

British troops entering an underground Maginot Line fortress in 1939

Did You Know?

Between 1929 and 1934, France built one of the strongest fortification systems in the world to protect its border from German invasion. The "Maginot Line" was a complex system of forts and barricades manned by thousands of **troops**. Later, Germans simply flew planes over it and sent troops around it.

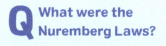

Q **What were the Nuremberg Laws?**

A In 1935, Germany enacted the "Nuremberg Laws." These laws stripped rights from Jewish citizens and allowed Nazi supporters to abuse them without fear of legal consequences.

TRUE OR FALSE?

Germany's **annexations** of Austria and part of Czechoslovakia in 1938 began the European war.

MOSTLY FALSE.

Although backed by threats of military force, the annexations were nonviolent occupations of German-speaking territories that Hitler claimed as part of "greater Germany." The fighting didn't start until Germany invaded Poland in September 1939.

Q **What was the Lend-Lease Act?**

A This was a US program launched in early 1941 to help Great Britain—and later other Allies—without violating the United States' official neutrality laws. Under the act, the United States lent $50 billion (about $575 billion today) worth of military equipment and supplies, including ships and tanks, to the Allies.

THE AXIS AND THE ALLIES

Q Who were the Allies?

A The Allies were nations that joined together to fight Germany, Japan, and other Axis countries. Leading members included the United Kingdom, the United States, and the Soviet Union.

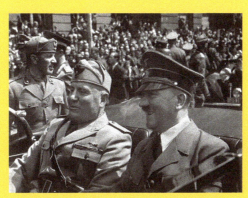

Mussolini (left) and Hitler in June 1940

Q What was the Axis?

A The Axis was a name coined by Italy's leader, Benito Mussolini. It was the alliance created in May 1939 between Germany and Italy. In September 1940, Japan joined as well. Other Axis nations included Albania, Bulgaria, Hungary, Romania, and Thailand.

Q Did the Allies include countries outside Europe?

A Yes. Argentina, Australia, Canada, China, Iran, Iraq, Mexico, New Zealand, South Africa, and Turkey all joined. Only Australia, Canada, China, and New Zealand were fully engaged in the war from start to finish, however.

Q Were the two sides in World War II the same as the sides in World War I?

A No. The main difference was that Italy and Japan fought with the Allies in the earlier war. Many countries that fought in the second war were not involved in the first war.

Q Did any major European nations remain **neutral** throughout the war?

A Ireland, Portugal, Spain, Sweden, and Switzerland remained neutral. Being "neutral" meant that they could profit by trading with both sides, but they had to remain ready to defend their neutrality should either side turn against them.

TRUE OR FALSE?

Some countries changed sides during the war.

TRUE.

None of the Allies changed sides, but several Axis members did. The most important Axis quitter was Italy, which surrendered to the Allies in September 1943 and then joined them.

Q **What part did Canada play in the war?**

A **One of the first Allied nations to declare war on Germany in September 1939, Canada fought hard in every major theater of the war and saw more than 100,000 of its people killed, wounded, or taken prisoner.**

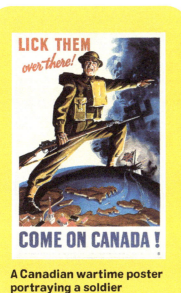

A Canadian wartime poster portraying a soldier

TRUE OR FALSE?

No Latin American countries fought in the war.

FALSE.

After declaring war on the Axis in early 1942, Mexico gave significant economic support to the Allies. It also lent troops to the US forces. Many other Latin American countries declared war on the Axis, but Brazil was the only other one to send troops and ships to fight.

TRUE OR FALSE?

*Adolf Hitler became **dictator** of Germany legally.*

TRUE.

Hitler was head of the Nazi Party during Germany's 1933 national elections. The party won the most seats in the legislature, known as the Reichstag. President Paul von Hindenburg appointed Hitler chancellor, making him the effective ruler of the country, which gave the Nazi Party power to form a government. Hitler then moved swiftly to increase his power. After Hindenburg died in 1934, Hitler became Germany's unchallenged dictator.

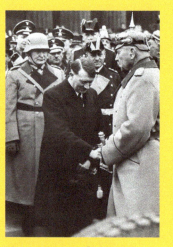

Hitler bows to German president Paul von Hindenburg in 1933

TRUE OR FALSE?

Hitler wasn't a natural-born German.

TRUE.

Born in the Austro-Hungarian Empire in 1889, Hitler renounced his Austrian citizenship in 1925 but didn't become a German citizen until 1932—the year before he became chancellor of Germany.

Q Who were the Nazis?

A The Nazis were members of Hitler's National Socialist Party, which ruled Germany from 1933 through the end of the war.

Q Where did the word "Nazi" come from?

A "Nazi" combines the first two letters of "national" with the second syllable of "sozialist" in "Nationalsozialistische Deutsche Arbeiterpartei," German for "National Socialist German Workers' Party." A German writer coined the term during the 1920s, when party members called themselves "Nasos." Because the word "Nazi" was similar to a Bavarian slang term for "simpleton," it caught on among party opponents. Party members themselves never used it.

TRUE OR FALSE?

All Germans were Nazis.

FALSE.

Nazis were card-carrying members of the National Socialist Party. They accounted for only about 10 percent of all Germans, but many other Germans supported the party.

Q Was the Nazi Party fascist?

A If **fascism** is defined broadly as a system of strong government and extreme **nationalism**, the answer is yes. Defined narrowly, the answer is probably no. Nazi Germany differed from fascist states like Italy, Spain, and Portugal in being even more nationalistic, more anti-church, and more dictatorial.

Q What is a swastika?

A An ancient symbol in many world cultures, including those of some Native Americans, the swastika is a cross whose arms are bent at 90-degree angles. The Nazi Party adopted it as its own and made it the official symbol of the Third Reich in 1935.

TRUE OR FALSE?

In 1939, America's Time *magazine named Adolf Hitler its "Man of the Year" for 1938—the same year Hitler had Germany occupy Austria and Czechoslovakia.*

TRUE.

However, Time's *publisher pointed out that the label was not meant to be an honor, but rather "a distinction applied to the newsmaker who most influenced world events for better or worse." Other wartime leaders* Time *designated Man of the Year included Franklin D. Roosevelt, Joseph Stalin, Winston Churchill, George Marshall, Dwight Eisenhower, and Harry Truman.*

A German general Erwin Rommel, who was noted for his clever tactics while commanding German troops in North Africa from 1941 to 1942, was known as "Desert Fox." However, he was badly defeated at El Alamein in Egypt. The British general who outfoxed him, Bernard Montgomery, was later given the title "Montgomery of Alamein."

Did You Know?

Benito Mussolini was named after 19th-century Mexican president Benito Juárez. Mussolini's father was a socialist who admired the Mexican hero for driving the French out of his country.

Did You Know?

Adolph Hitler and Franklin D. Roosevelt were in power at almost exactly the same time. Hitler became Germany's chancellor on January 30, 1933. Roosevelt became the US president 33 days later. Roosevelt died on April 12, 1945. Hitler died by suicide 18 days later.

Q What kind of government did Japan have?

A Like Great Britain, Japan was a monarchy with an elected parliament before the war. It gave a little more power to its emperor, Hirohito, but gradually allowed its military to control the government.

Q What was Emperor Hirohito's role in the war?

A Hirohito's power was more symbolic than real. It is not known exactly how much influence he had during the war. However, while he apparently did not push for war, he did little to stop it until the very end.

Q If Emperor Hirohito didn't really rule Japan, who did?

A General Hideki Tojo was the most powerful leader in government. As the war progressed, he increased his powers until he was virtually a dictator.

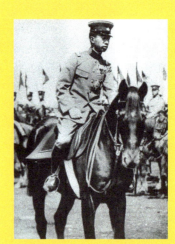

Emperor Hirohito rides in a military parade during the 1930s

Q Who were Tokyo Rose and Axis Sally?

A These were popular nicknames for women who broadcast **propaganda** to US troops from Japan and Germany in order to lower morale. The American woman best known as "Tokyo Rose," Iva Toguri D'Aquino, was convicted of treason and imprisoned after the war.

Q Did Japanese and German propaganda broadcasts actually damage morale among American soldiers and sailors?

A Probably not. Homesick troops enjoyed the popular American music the broadcasts played and generally laughed off the obviously untrue propaganda.

Q Which country had the best spies?

A No one really knows. All countries in the war used spies for valuable work, but because of the secrecy and lying connected with spying, it is nearly impossible to separate fact from fiction.

TRUE OR FALSE?

Russia and the Soviet Union were the same country.

FALSE.

After the 1917 Russian Revolution overthrew the old Russian Empire, a new kind of empire rose under the dictatorial rule of the Communist Party. It called itself the "Union of Soviet Socialist Republics" (USSR), or "Soviet Union," and joined Russia with many of its neighbors as individual "republics" within the union. Although Russia was the largest and most influential of these new republics, it remained distinct from the others. Russian was the USSR's official language, but not all Soviet people were Russian.

Q **What kind of government did the Soviet Union have?**

A **The Russian Revolution led to the creation of a dictatorial communist government that controlled almost every aspect of the economy and people's lives. As head of the Communist Party, Joseph Stalin was a ruthless dictator who wanted to increase his own power and to defeat Germany.**

Q **Was Stalin really not a Russian?**

A **Stalin was born in what is now the nation of Georgia, which had originally been an independent kingdom. When Stalin was born there in 1878, Georgia was part of the Russian Empire, and it later became part of the Soviet Union, just as Russia itself was.**

Q Was the Soviet Union allied with the Western democracies even though it had a different type of government?

A Yes. The one thing all the Allies agreed about was the need to defeat Nazi Germany. Stalin surprised the Allies by signing a friendship treaty with Germany in 1939, hoping it would keep Germany from invading the Soviet Union while Soviet forces grew stronger. Then, Hitler surprised Stalin by invading anyway in 1941.

Q Did the Soviet Union also fight against Japan in the Pacific War?

A Yes, but only briefly. The two countries clashed in China in 1939 but signed a neutrality pact two years later. They didn't meet again in battle until after Germany had surrendered and the United States had dropped its first **atomic bomb** on Japan in August 1945.

Q Did women hold leadership positions in any major Allied or Axis government?

A No. The war opened employment and **military auxiliary** opportunities for millions of women, but no women rose to top-level positions in any government or military force.

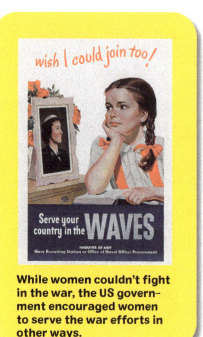

wish I could join too!

Serve your country in the **WAVES**

INQUIRE AT ANY
Navy Recruiting Station or Office of Naval Officer Procurement

While women couldn't fight in the war, the US government encouraged women to serve the war efforts in other ways.

NUMBER OF PEOPLE IN EACH COUNTRY'S MILITARY

China	14 million
France	3.5 million
Germany	9.5 million
Italy	9 million
Japan	9.1 million
Poland	2.4 million
Soviet Union	21 million
United States	16.35 million
United Kingdom	5.9 million

PEOPLE, WEAPONS, AND TOOLS OF WAR

Q What were the biggest differences between World War II weapons and those of earlier wars?

A Guns, ships, tanks, and airplanes were bigger, faster, and stronger. Better tanks made armies more mobile. Better planes made aerial bombings more widespread and deadlier, and navies fought more with airplanes than with their ships' big guns. **Radar**, helicopters, jet planes, big rocket bombs, and atomic bombs were also new to warfare.

TRUE OR FALSE?

Aircraft carriers were more important than battleships in the war.

TRUE.

Most Pacific sea battles pitted planes against ships, and carriers could transport planes over distances land-based planes couldn't reach. Battleships helped by escorting carriers and bombarding enemies on land. The United States stopped making battleships during the war, and hasn't made one since. Aircraft carriers played a smaller role in the Atlantic war. Germany started to build some but never completed any.

Q How important were submarines?

A Submarines were very important. German subs devastated Allied shipping in the Atlantic, and Japanese subs did the same in the Pacific. Eventually, however, the Allies destroyed most enemy subs and used their own subs to target Axis shipping.

Stat: US submarines operated mostly in the Pacific, where they sank almost **1,300** Japanese merchant ships, **8** aircraft carriers, **1** battleship, **12** cruisers, **42** destroyers, and **22** subs.

Did You Know?

World War II was the first war in which antibiotics were used to treat wounded soldiers. Discovered in 1928, penicillin saved so many Allied lives that it was called a "miracle drug." After the war, it changed modern medicine.

Myth:

By the time the war ended, Germany was close to developing its own atomic bomb.

Truth:

Germany had many top scientists working on a nuclear weapon. However, they never achieved the chain reaction necessary to make a bomb work. Germany gave up on its project before the war ended.

Stat: Animals also played important roles through-out the war. The US Army's Quartermaster Corps, for example, trained **10,425** dogs to serve as sentries, scouts, patrols, messengers, and land-mine detectors.

Q **What exactly are tanks?**

A Tanks are heavily armed and armored land vehicles whose caterpillar treads let them move rapidly over all types of terrain. Invented during World War I, they became the most important assault vehicles of World War II, which employed hundreds of thousands of them. The United States' famous Sherman tank was the best Allied tank. Almost 50,000 were produced. They served in every theater of the war. Even the Soviet army used Sherman tanks.

Q **What's a bazooka?**

A A bazooka is a handheld rocket launcher that fires projectiles heavy enough to break through thick armor. The United States developed bazookas to give infantry soldiers weapons that could stop enemy tanks.

TRUE OR FALSE?

Jet fighter planes fought during the war.

TRUE.

Germany, Japan, Great Britain, the United States, and the Soviet Union all developed jets before the war ended, but only German and British fighter jets saw much combat action.

- -

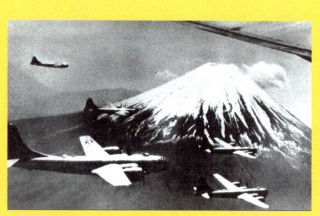

B-29s flying past Mt. Fuji on their way to Tokyo

Q What was the war's most advanced bomber?

A The Boeing B-29 Superfortress had the greatest range and carried the heaviest bomb loads. It was also fast, well-armored, and able to fly so high that enemy fighters and anti-aircraft guns had trouble reaching it.

Stat: Although not introduced to the war until mid-1944, more than **3,000** B-29 bombers flew **34,790 sorties**, dropped **170,000** tons of bombs—including both atomic bombs—on Japan, and shot down **1,128** enemy planes.

Q What made the Japanese Zero such a dangerous fighter plane?

A In 1941, it was the fastest and most agile plane fighting in the Pacific. Well-armed and able to climb rapidly, it could fly circles around Allied planes. As US fighter planes improved, however, it lost its advantages. Many Zeros ended the war as **kamikaze** suicide bombs.

Did You Know?

The Japanese company that built the Zero was part of the same parent company that makes modern Mitsubishi automobiles.

Did You Know?

Giant airships were important in World War I, but the only airships in World War II were smaller US Navy blimps. Blimps proved so useful for detecting enemy submarines that the Navy increased their number from 10 to 167 by the end of the war. No **convoy** escorted by a blimp ever lost a ship to enemy action.

Who were the Navajo code talkers?

A About 300 Native Americans served in the Marine Corps as radio operators in the Pacific. They were known as the Navajo code talkers because by using their own language, they exchanged military messages the Japanese could never figure out.

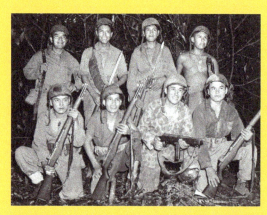

Navajo code talkers on a South Pacific island

TRUE OR FALSE?

Radar helped the Allies win the war.

TRUE.

Radar is an electronic system for detecting and tracking distant objects, such as ships and aircraft. It was developed by American and British scientists and used by the Allied nations before the Axis nations had it. Having radar early on helped the British to win the Battle of Britain and the United States to win early naval battles with Japan.

Q What was
Operation Magic?

A Operation Magic was a program the United States
started before the war. Its purpose was to break
codes that Japan used in secret radio messages. It
only partly succeeded before the Pearl Harbor attack,
but soon became so advanced that the United States
used decoded messages to help win important battles.

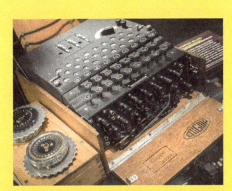

The Enigma machine was used to
code and decode messages.

Q What was Germany's
Enigma machine?

A Germany's Enigma machine was a complicated
device for coding and decoding radio messages.
Germany used it to transmit secret messages between
military units. Thanks to the Polish government's
interception of a manual for an Enigma machine, the
British were able to build their own to decode German
messages, giving the Allies a huge advantage.

TRUE OR FALSE?

The US Army and Navy were racially segregated during the war.

TRUE.

Black and Japanese American servicemen had to train, live, serve, and fight in units apart from those of white Americans. Racial segregation in the military did not officially end until President Harry Truman issued an executive order outlawing it in July 1948.

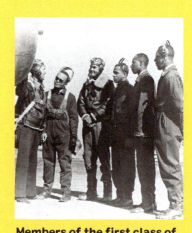

Members of the first class of Tuskegee Airman (Benjamin O. Davis is third from left).

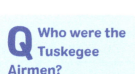

Q Who were the Tuskegee Airmen?

A The Tuskegee Airmen were pilots in an African American Army Air Corps unit who trained at the Tuskegee Institute, the Alabama college for Black students founded by Booker T. Washington. Initially denied combat roles in the segregated Army, the Black pilots eventually proved their worth by shooting down 261 enemy planes, winning more than 850 medals, and becoming one of the most distinguished fighter groups of the war.

Q Did Latinos serve in racially segregated military units?

A Puerto Ricans did, but other American Latinos served alongside white soldiers and sailors.

Did You Know?

The only Black general in the US Army during the war was Benjamin O. Davis. His son, Benjamin O. Davis Jr., commanded the Tuskegee Airmen and later became the first Black general in the US Air Force.

Q Did women serve in the US military?

A In early 1942, the Army created an auxiliary corps for women, but soon gave it full military status as the Women's Army Corps (WAC). The Navy created the Women Accepted for Volunteer Emergency Service (WAVES), the Coast Guard the SPARs (short for the Coast Guard motto, "Semper Paratus," meaning "always ready"), and the Marines the Women's Reserve. About 350,000 women served in these branches, performing mainly noncombat work that otherwise would have been done by male servicemen.

Q Who were the Flying Tigers?

A The "Flying Tigers" were a group of about 100 American volunteers who flew P-40 fighter planes provided by the US government for the Republic of China between 1941 and 1942. The noses of their planes were decorated with menacing shark's teeth and eyes.

Q Were poison gases used in combat as much in World War II as they had been in World War I?

A No. The Japanese used gas in China in 1941, and the Italians used gas in Ethiopia in 1936. Otherwise, countries honored the Geneva Convention rule against using poison gas. Nevertheless, all sides were prepared to defend against possible gas attacks.

Q How were glider planes used in the war?

A Towed by powered planes, gliders landed jeeps, artillery weapons, and as many as 40 troops at a time behind enemy lines. The Germans were the first to use gliders but lost interest in them. Meanwhile, the Allies borrowed the idea from the Germans and made great use of gliders. The United States alone made more than 13,000 glider planes. Each plane was normally used just once.

TRUE OR FALSE?

The US Coast Guard didn't fight in the war.

FALSE.

Although normally an independent service, the Coast Guard operated in the war as a branch of the Navy. It specialized in dangerous rescues and small-boat operations, protecting ports, and patrolling shorelines.

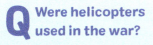

Q **Were helicopters used in the war?**

A **Yes. Several nations, including the United States, started developing helicopters and their close cousins, autogiros, as the war began. Only small numbers saw military service, mainly in submarine detection and rescue operations.**

TRUE OR FALSE?

Horse-riding cavalry soldiers played important roles in the war.

MOSTLY FALSE.

*By the time the war started, tanks had replaced horses in most armies, though a few—particularly the Soviet **Red Army**—still had mounted cavalry units. Horses were also still used for pulling artillery and carrying supplies, especially by the Germans.*

A The 34th president, Dwight D. Eisenhower,
served as supreme Allied commander in Europe.
The president after Eisenhower, John F. Kennedy,
commanded Navy patrol boats in the Pacific. Lyndon
B. Johnson, Gerald Ford, and George H. W. Bush also
served in the Navy in the Pacific. Future presidents
who served on the home front included Richard Nixon
and Ronald Reagan. Jimmy Carter was at the Naval
Academy during the war.

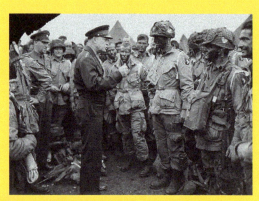

General Eisenhower encouraging Allied
paratroopers on the eve of D-Day

Did You Know?

Future president John F. Kennedy commanded a
patrol boat (PT-109) in the Solomon Islands that was
rammed and sunk by a Japanese destroyer in 1943.
He saved fellow crewmen's lives, earning medals
for heroism.

Did You Know?

The US Air Force was not an independent service until 1947. Throughout the war, it was known as the "US Army Air Forces" (USAAF), and was under the command of the US Army.

Stat: During the war, the USAAF added **229,554** new aircraft of all types. The Navy added more than **75,000** aircraft, mostly combat fighters.

Q Where did the expression "G.I. Joe" come from?

A A good-natured nickname for the typical American soldier, it first appeared in an Army magazine comic strip in 1942. "G.I." stood for "government issue," a military phrase suggesting "average."

MANY US NAVY SHIPS WERE NAMED AFTER PEOPLE, PLACES, AND THINGS IN DIFFERENT CATEGORIES.

CLASS	CATEGORY	EXAMPLES
Battleships	US states	*Arizona, Missouri*
Aircraft carriers	Historic battles and ships	*Lexington, Yorktown*
Cruisers	Cities	*Indianapolis, Los Angeles*
Destroyers	Distinguished Navy and Marine veterans	*The Sullivans*
Submarines	Sea creatures	*Gato, Swordfish*

BATTLES OF THE WAR

Q What happened at Dunkirk?

A Dunkirk is a northern French seaport where 338,000 British, French, and Belgian troops were trapped by the Germans in late May 1940. Their situation looked hopeless, but thanks to 1,200 naval and **civilian** vessels, nearly all the Allied troops were evacuated to Britain by early June.

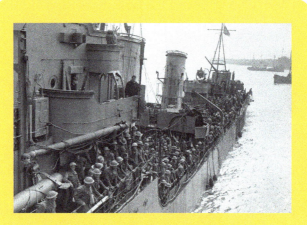

British troops being evacuated from Dunkirk

Did You Know?

The four-day Battle of the Coral Sea in May 1942 was the first major battle between the US and Japanese navies. It was also history's first naval battle in which enemy ships never even saw each other. All the fighting involved planes from aircraft carriers.

Q Why was the tiny Pacific island of Midway the center of such an important battle?

A Midway was a US Navy base the Japanese wanted for themselves. In June 1942, Japan launched a huge air-and-sea attack, hoping to complete the destruction of America's Pacific **Fleet**. By decoding Japanese messages, the United States figured out Japan's plans and not only won the battle but also sank four aircraft carriers, weakening Japan's navy through the rest of the war.

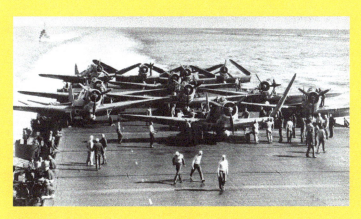

US Navy planes preparing to fight in the Battle of Midway

Stat: The most dangerous type of duty during the war was submarine service. The United States lost **22 percent** of its subs, Italy **33 percent**, Japan more than **50 percent**, and Germany at least **70 percent**. Unlike surface vessels, when subs sank they usually went down with their entire crews.

Q What kind of battle was the Battle of Britain?

A The Battle of Britain was a long-running aerial battle between Germany's **Luftwaffe** and Britain's Royal Air Force (**RAF**). They fought over southern England from July to October 1940. Germany hoped to destroy the RAF to make invasion of Britain possible, but thanks to radar warnings, RAF planes won despite being badly outnumbered.

TRUE OR FALSE?

The Blitz was another name for the Battle of Britain.

PARTLY TRUE.

The Blitz was the second phase of the Battle of Britain, when Germany switched to heavily bombing London and other English cities in night raids. The raids killed thousands of civilians and caused heavy damage but didn't greatly hurt Britain's war efforts.

Did You Know?

Despite being in one of London's most heavily bombed areas, St. Paul's Cathedral survived with only minor damage.

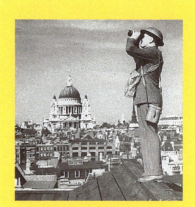

A London aircraft spotter watching for German bombers near St. Paul's Cathedral

Did You Know?

Japan's surprise attack on Pearl Harbor in Hawaii on December 7, 1941, began *before* its airplanes arrived there. Several hours earlier, the Japanese navy launched five mini submarines toward the harbor. Each had a two-man crew and carried two torpedoes. A US destroyer sank the first sub before any Japanese planes were even seen. Four of the five subs were sunk, and the fifth ran aground.

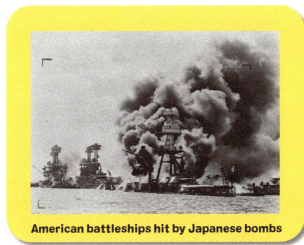

American battleships hit by Japanese bombs

Myth:

President Roosevelt knew in advance that the Pearl Harbor attack was coming but did nothing to stop it so that public anger against Japan would support US entry into the war.

Truth:

Roosevelt learned enough from intercepted Japanese communications to know that US bases in Guam and the Philippines were threatened, and he made sure military commanders were warned. However, he was as surprised as everyone else when the Japanese attacked Pearl Harbor.

Stat: Japan's Pearl Harbor attack sank **6** battleships, **3** cruisers, and **4** smaller vessels. It also damaged **2** other battleships, and destroyed **188** US aircraft, killing **2,403** military personnel and civilians. The Japanese lost **29** planes, **1** major submarine, and **5** mini submarines.

Q Was Japan's attack on Pearl Harbor a success?

A Yes and no. The raid severely damaged US warships and planes, and Japanese losses were small. However, the raid did not touch American aircraft carriers that would later help defeat Japan's navy. Plus, most of the damaged US warships were repaired and put back into service. More importantly, the raid unified US public opinion against Japan, ensuring that the United States would do everything it could to defeat Japan.

Myth:
Some Japanese Americans living in Hawaii helped the Japanese attack by acting as spies.

Truth:
There's not a single documented case of any Japanese Americans helping Japan in the attack.

Q What was the
Phony War?

A The "Phony War" was the seven-month period
starting September 3, 1939, when Germany invaded
Poland, and France and Great Britain declared war.
It went on until April 9, 1940, when Germany invaded
Norway and Denmark. Although France and Great
Britain expected to be attacked, almost nothing
happened between those dates.

Q What was the war's most
devastating battle?

A The Battle of Stalingrad (present-day Volgograd)
in southern Russia was probably the most
devastating. Between August 1942 and February 1943,
a German army nearly destroyed the city, but heavy
Soviet resistance eventually forced the Germans to
surrender. About 268,000 German soldiers were killed,
wounded, or captured, and about one million Soviet
soldiers and civilians were killed. The battle ended
Hitler's hopes of conquering the Soviet Union.

Did You Know?

Thanks to the work of code breakers, US Navy fighter planes intercepted and shot down the plane carrying Japan's top naval commander, Admiral Isoroku Yamamoto, on a tour of island bases in April 1943. Yamamoto's death dealt a serious blow to Japan's operations in the Pacific. The United States kept details of the operation secret until after the war ended.

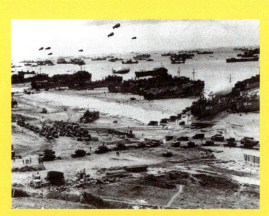

Allies landing troops and supplies on Omaha Beach on D-Day

Q What was D-Day?

A D-Day occurred on June 6, 1944, when the Allies began the invasion of Europe by landing massive forces along the beaches of Normandy on France's northern coast. Perhaps the single most important turning point of the war, the day marked the beginning of the end for Nazi Germany.

Stat: More than two and a half years in its planning, the D-Day invasion involved **154,000** British, Canadian, and American troops. It used **13,175** aircraft, **5,000** ships, **20,000** land vehicles, and **347** minesweepers. It sailed the largest armada ever gathered in world history.

Did You Know?

As many as 300,000 French **Resistance** fighters **sabotaged** German operations, collected information for the Allies, killed collaborators, and even fought German soldiers. Their activities greatly helped the Allied invasion after D-Day.

Q How did the Battle of the Bulge get its odd name?

A The "Bulge" was not a place but a big bend, or "bulge," in the German lines, when a sudden German offensive in December 1944 surprised Allied forces in Belgium. It was Hitler's last-gasp effort to stop an Allied invasion of Germany itself. The Battle of the Bulge inflicted huge losses on both sides, but opened western approaches to Germany and weakened Germany's ability to resist the Soviet invasion in the east.

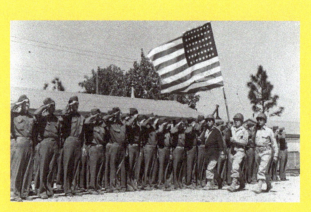

Members of the 442nd Regimental Combat Team

Q What was the most highly decorated US combat unit, not only in the war, but also in US military history?

A The 442nd Regimental Combat Team, made up of Japanese American troops, fought in Italy and France. Its members earned more than 18,000 individual decorations, and the team earned four Distinguished Unit Citations for extraordinary heroism.

Q Why did Germany fight in far-off North Africa?

A It fought there primarily to challenge British control of routes to Middle Eastern oil sources and the Suez Canal. But after a great German defeat in Egypt, Hitler turned his attention back to Europe.

Stat: Toward the end of the Pacific War, as its losing efforts became more desperate, Japan sent **2,393** untrained kamikaze pilots to die, directed to fly planes loaded with explosives directly into Allied warships. 34 ships sank, but because the pilots weren't trained, most kamikaze planes were shot down.

Stat: Allied bombs and torpedoes sank at least **16** Japanese ships carrying Allied prisoners of war, unknowingly killing more than **20,000** fellow Allies.

Stat: The five-week-long Battle of Iwo Jima in early 1945 had the highest mortality rate for one side of any major battle in the war. Of the **23,000** Japanese soldiers defending the small island against far more numerous American troops, fewer than **230** (**1 percent**) survived.

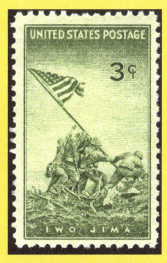

A US postage stamp issued in 1945, showing Marines raising the flag on Iwo Jima

LIFE ON THE HOME FRONTS

Stat: World War II had a high civilian death rate. In the US Civil War, only about **7 percent** of the deaths were civilians. In World War I, the figure was about **20 percent**. In World War II, that figure jumped to almost **60 percent**. Reasons included disease, starvation, heavy bombing, and **genocide**.

Did You Know?

Throughout Europe, children were evacuated from combat and bombing zones, and many became orphans and **refugees**. In Britain alone, more than one million children were evacuated to rural towns from London and other cities. Some went to the United States, Canada, and other countries. In contrast, when German cities began suffering heavy bombing, Hitler was reluctant to allow mass evacuations, so many German children died who might have been saved.

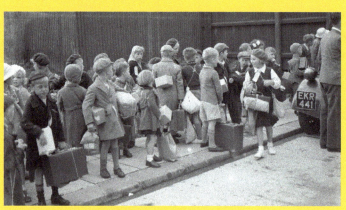

English children being evacuated from a city

TRUE OR FALSE?

*Most nations fighting in the war introduced **rationing** systems.*

TRUE.

As wartime needs caused food and other shortages, governments instituted increasingly tough rationing rules. Great Britain, for example, issued ration cards to every man, woman, and child, limiting purchases of meat, milk, eggs, butter, cheese, and sugar. Germany had similar systems for itself and countries it occupied, but didn't share goods evenly.

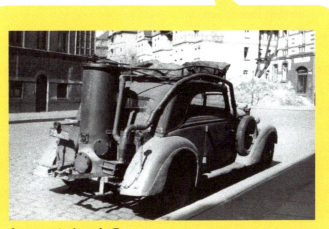

A converted car in Europe

Stat: During the war years, Japan and European countries had so little gasoline they modified a million cars and other vehicles to burn wood and charcoal for fuel. By the end of the war, Germany alone had **500,000** such vehicles.

Q What was the Holocaust?

A The Holocaust refers to Nazi Germany's efforts to kill all European Jews. That terrible plan wasn't a vague idea; it was shockingly real. During Hitler's years in power, German authorities ordered the killing of at least six million Jews, along with many other people the Nazis deemed "undesirable," such as Romanis and LGBTQ people.

Q Which occupied country did the Germans treat most harshly?

A Germany's six-year occupation of Poland was a terrifying nightmare. The Germans drove Poles from their homes, worked them to death in labor camps, murdered their leaders, and killed almost all the country's millions of Jews in death camps.

ESTIMATED JEWISH DEATHS IN THE COUNTRIES HARDEST HIT BY THE HOLOCAUST

Poland	3,000,000
Soviet Union	700,00–1,340,000
Hungary	400,000–550,000
Romania	230,000–271,000
Czechoslovakia	149,200–310,000
Estonia, Latvia, and Lithuania	200,000
Germany	135,000–330,000
Netherlands	100,000–117,000
France	75,000–120,000

Q Who was Anne Frank (1929–1945)?

A Anne Frank was a Jewish German girl who hid from the Nazis for nearly two years with her family and some friends in an Amsterdam house. She was eventually captured and died in a concentration camp. Her diary was published after the war, making her famous as a symbol of courage and faith in humanity.

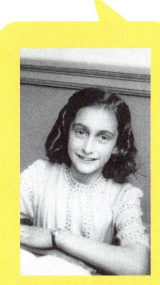

Anne Frank smiles for a school photograph.

Q Were German concentration camps the same as prisoner of war (POW) camps?

A No. POW camps held Allied servicemen in conditions reasonably in accord with Geneva Convention standards. Concentration camps held mostly civilian men, women, and children—including Jews, Romani people, people with mental health problems, political opponents, and other so-called "undesirables." Conditions were so terrible that many prisoners died of starvation, disease, and cold weather. In many camps, Nazis killed prisoners with poison gas.

What was life like for ordinary Japanese citizens as the war waged on?

A As most Japanese merchant ships were sunk, people at home suffered growing shortages of food and fuel. Meanwhile, Allied air-bombing raids devastated Japanese cities.

Did You Know?

The war's single most destructive bombing attack was not one of the atomic bombings but the Allied firebombing of Tokyo on March 9, 1945. Nearly 300 B-29s dropped 2,000 tons of incendiary bombs that burned down a quarter of the capital city's buildings, killing around 100,000 people, and leaving one million homeless. Emperor Hirohito's shock at the extent of the destruction contributed to his subesquent decision to surrender.

TRUE OR FALSE?

Children generally suffered less during the war than adult civilians.

FALSE.

Tens of millions of children lost their homes, were killed by disease, starved to death, were sent to concentration camps, or were otherwise separated from their parents or orphaned. In addition, almost all children in combat zones were badly traumatized.

Q How did children in the United States help in the war effort?

A US children bought defense stamps, joined Junior Red Cross programs, volunteered to do farm work, and assisted in scrap drives, which collected recyclable materials such as rubber tires and metals to help the war effort.

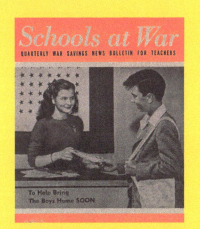

Schools at War was a federal government program created to involve American children in the war effort.

Q What were war bonds and defense stamps?

A These were loan certificates issued by the federal government to raise money for the war. Bonds were basically low-interest loans buyers made to the government. From late 1942 to the end of the war, the government raised $190 billion through bond drives. Movie stars and comic books played a big role in promoting their sales. Cheaper "defense stamps" were also sold, mainly to children.

Q How did rationing work in the United States?

A Every man, woman, and child received monthly coupons—and later "points"—to use for purchases.

Q What were black markets?

A Illegal markets selling goods to evade government restrictions were called "black markets." Food, fuel, and other goods were sold at inflated prices in black markets in most nations involved in the war.

Did You Know?

Because of wartime copper shortages, US pennies minted in 1943 were made of 99 percent steel, instead of copper. Those "steelies" are the only regular-issue US coins attracted by magnets.

Q Did members of the US armed forces pay to mail letters home?

A No. Under a War Powers Act, they were entitled to free postage.

Did You Know?

Japan's Pearl Harbor attack prompted the US government to commit a terrible violation of civil rights. In February 1942, President Roosevelt ordered the imprisonment of 120,000 people of Japanese descent living in West Coast states in "relocation" or "internment" camps for the duration of the war. Thousands of native-born American citizens lost their homes, farms, businesses, and freedom.

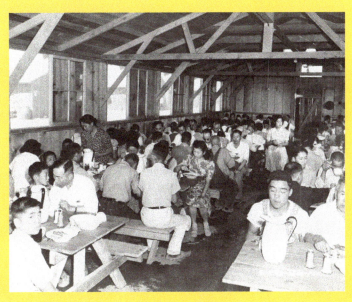

Japanese American families in the dining hall of the Pinedale, California, internment camp

Q How did the war change the roles of American women?

A As men left factory jobs for the military, many were replaced by women, most of whom previously hadn't done tough factory labor. Not only did women workers do well, but they often proved themselves to be better than men at doing factory work. As millions of women moved from administrative and retail jobs to factory work, they, in turn, were replaced by other women entering the workforce for the first time.

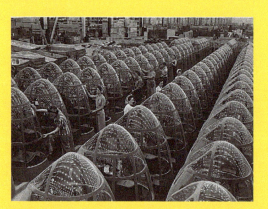

Women assembling bomber nose cones

Q Was Rosie the Riveter a real person?

A No. She was a symbolic figure created to encourage women in the United States to join in the war effort by taking on jobs traditionally restricted to men, such as building airplanes.

Q What was civil defense?

A "Civil defense" government programs prepared communities to assist in their own defense during enemy attacks. Given the unlikelihood of ground invasion, attention was focused on possible air raids. Millions of registered volunteers watched for enemy aircraft, neighborhoods prepared for emergencies, and citizens were encouraged to support scrap drives and war bond campaigns.

Q Did enemy troops ever land in the United States?

A Yes. From 1942 to 1943, Japanese troops briefly occupied two remote islands in the Aleutian chain in Alaska, which was then a US territory.

Q Were there other kinds of enemy attacks on the continental United States?

A Japanese submarines ineffectively shelled Pacific coastal areas in early 1942, and Japanese balloon bombs were sent to the United States toward the war's end. Those attacks did little damage.

Q What were
balloon bombs?

A From late 1944 through early 1945, Japan released more than 9,000 balloon bombs carrying explosive and fire-starting devices across the Pacific. The Japanese hoped the bombs would start wildfires, kill people, and cause panic. Many balloons reached the United States and Canada. One bomb killed six people in Oregon. Otherwise, they did little damage.

Q Did enemy propaganda have any impact on the American home front?

A Occasionally, yes. In 1945, the US Office of Censorship banned the publication of news about Japan's balloon bombs, but false Japanese reports of the bombs causing fires and deaths reached the United States. People panicked, and the government lifted its ban so that correct information could be published.

Q What were
Victory Gardens?

A US families planted food gardens, called "Victory Gardens," in their yards and public places. These gardens dealt with wartime food shortages. More than 20 million such gardens eventually produced 40 percent of all vegetables eaten on the home front.

A These were federal laws passed in December 1941 and March 1942 that gave the president and Interstate Commerce Commission sweeping powers over wartime production, prices, the distribution of goods, transportation, communications, and other matters. President Roosevelt used those powers to order the internment of Japanese Americans and to force the automobile industry to produce military vehicles and planes.

Did You Know?

In early 1942, the federal government shut down the production of civilian cars so automobile plants would instead make military vehicles and planes. No more civilian cars were made again until 1946.

Did You Know?

A great economic miracle of the war was the rapid expansion of the US aircraft industry. In 1939, the industry produced about 6,000 planes. Between 1940 and 1945, it produced 300,000 planes, making it the largest industry in the country.

Stat: Before the war, US shipping yards built only **15** naval vessels a year. During the war years, expanded shipyards working **24** hours a day increased that rate by **40** times to produce **6,500** naval vessels, **6,500** cargo ships, and **64,500** landing craft.

Did You Know?

After releasing *Bambi* in 1942, the Walt Disney Company made short films supporting Allied war efforts. Among its numerous propaganda films was *Der Fuehrer's Face*, a cartoon in which Donald Duck dreams about living in "Nutziland."

TRUE OR FALSE?

Comic books contributed to the US war effort.

TRUE.

Wartime comics about Superman, Wonder Woman, Captain America, and other superheroes constantly promoted patriotism and the need for young readers to buy war bonds and defense stamps. The biggest readers of comics, however, were not children, but troops serving in the war.

Q Were the Olympic Games held anywhere during the war?

A No. The 1940 games scheduled for Tokyo were canceled. The 1944 games scheduled for London were postponed until 1948.

Q How did the war affect US baseball?

A Most minor leagues shut down. Numerous major league players—including many big stars—enlisted in the military, but the majors kept operating by adding foreign and older players.

THE WAR'S END AND AFTERMATH

Q What were V–E Day and V–J Day?

A These were the dates when the Allies officially declared victories. "Victory in Europe" day was May 8, 1945. "Victory over Japan" day was August 14, 1945.

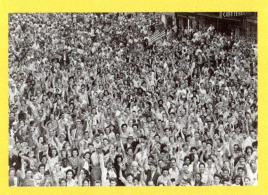

Americans celebrating the end of the war in New York's Times Square

Q How many assassination attempts were made on Hitler?

A At least three. In late 1939, a bomb exploded after he left a Munich building. In March 1943, German army officers placed a bomb in his plane, but it failed to go off. In July 1944, another bomb just missed killing him.

Q What strange stunt to end the war with Great Britain did Hitler's trusted deputy Rudolf Hess try?

A Without telling anyone his plans, Hess flew a plane to Scotland in 1941, hoping to open peace negotiations with the British. He was instead taken prisoner, and Hitler denounced him as crazy. Hess remained a prisoner for the rest of his long life.

Q How did the European war end in Germany?

A With Allied armies closing in on Berlin in April 1945, Hitler wouldn't consider an orderly surrender and instead died by suicide, allowing Germany to collapse around him.

Did You Know?

Before Hitler died on April 30, 1945, he named Grand Admiral Karl Dönitz his successor as chancellor. Dönitz held the post long enough to negotiate Germany's surrender on May 7. The Allies then arrested him and convicted him of **war crimes** at the Nuremberg Trials.

TRUE OR FALSE?

Italy surrendered to the Allies almost two years before Germany did.

MOSTLY TRUE.

Political rivals ousted Mussolini in July 1943. Two months later, the new government surrendered to the invading Allied armies and declared war on Germany. Meanwhile, German troops rescued Mussolini and helped him set up a puppet government in northern Italy.

Did You Know?

Franklin Roosevelt, Benito Mussolini, and Adolf Hitler all died within one three-week period in April 1945. Roosevelt died of natural causes on April 12, Mussolini was assassinated on April 28, and Hitler died by suicide on April 30.

Stat: According to National World War II Museum estimates, the war killed at least **70 million** people worldwide. About **25 million** deaths were military personnel, and the rest were civilians. China and the Soviet Union suffered the greatest losses, with at least **20 million** deaths each. Other countries with terrible death tolls included Germany (**8.8 million**), Poland (**5.6 million**), Japan (**3.1 million**), India (**2.5 million**), the Philippines (**1 million**), Romania (**833,000**), Greece (**800,000**), Hungary (**580,000**), France (**567,000**), Italy (**457,000**), the United Kingdom (**451,000**), and the United States (**418,000**).

Myth:

Japan was already prepared to surrender before the atomic bombs were dropped on Hiroshima and Nagasaki in August 1945.

Truth:

Japan wasn't quick to surrender, even after the second atomic bomb destroyed Nagasaki. It took the Soviet declaration of war and another bombing raid on Tokyo to cause Japan to surrender. Without the atomic bombs, Japan's surrender might have come much later.

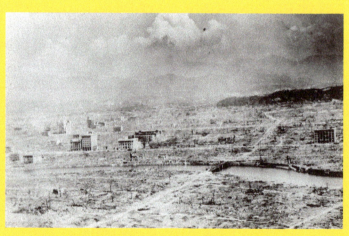

Hiroshima after the atomic bomb blast

Did You Know?

The code names for the atomic bombs dropped on Japan were "Little Boy" and "Fat Man," but Little Boy was originally called "Thin Man" because it was thinner than Fat Man.

Did You Know?

When Japan broadcast Hirohito's speech announcing Japan's surrender to the Allies on August 15, 1945, it was the first time ordinary Japanese citizens had heard any emperor's voice.

Q **What were the Nuremberg Trials?**

A The Nuremberg Trials were a series of trials of German government and military officers charged with war crimes. Conducted by the Allies, the trials were held in Nuremberg, Germany. The first one tried 21 top leaders, including Hermann Göring, Rudolf Hess, Joachim von Ribbentrop, and Karl Dönitz. Twelve defendants were condemned to death, seven were sentenced to prison, and three were acquitted. Lower-level officials were prosecuted in 12 later trials.

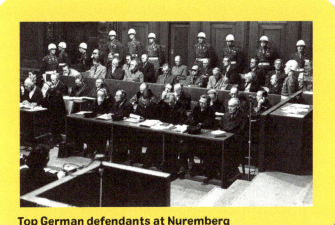

Top German defendants at Nuremberg

Did You Know?

Seven German leaders convicted at Nuremberg were sent to Berlin's Spandau Prison. By 1966, the only one still there was Rudolf Hess. He remained the only inmate until his death in 1987.

Q Are Nazi war criminals still being hunted around the world?

A Yes. As recently as 2021, the United States deported a 95-year-old man to Germany. He had been a concentration camp guard toward the end of the war. He had been living in the United States for more than 70 years.

TRUE OR FALSE?

The Allies' war-crimes trials in Japan were even bigger than those in Germany.

TRUE.

Between 1946 and 1948, about 5,600 Japanese military and government leaders were tried in Tokyo, primarily for their atrocities against Allied prisoners of war and civilians in occupied countries. Almost 4,000 defendants were convicted and 1,000 were executed, including former prime minister Hideki Tojo.

A Hirohito himself expected to be tried and executed, but the United States decided not to try him so he could remain a stabilizing, though powerless, force in Japanese government and society.

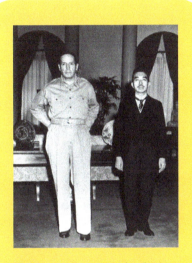

US general Douglas MacArthur (left) with Japanese emperor Hirohito. After the war, MacArthur was named supreme Allied commander of Japan.

TRUE OR FALSE?

Dozens of Japanese soldiers stayed hidden on Pacific islands decades after the war ended.

TRUE.

Some holdouts didn't know the war had ended. Others didn't believe it or refused to accept Japan's surrender. The last-known holdout was found in 1974.

- - - - - - - - - - - - - - -

Q What became of the
League of Nations?

A With its reputation as a peacekeeping organization ruined by its failure to prevent international crises, it gradually lost members until it was replaced by the new United Nations as the war was ending.

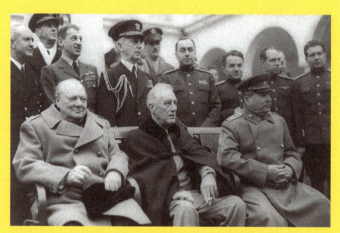

British prime minister Winston Churchill (left), US president Franklin Roosevelt, and Soviet premier Joseph Stalin at Yalta in early 1945

Q How did the war change the map of Europe?

A Germany's defeat restored the independence of countries it had occupied, and some border adjustments were made. Germany itself was divided between the Federal Republic of (West) Germany and the Democratic Republic of (East) Germany. Berlin, although inside East Germany, was also divided. In Eastern Europe, the Soviet Union made East Germany, Poland, Czechoslovakia, and other countries its satellites, or junior partners. Germany finally reunified in 1990.

Q Did the war change the maps of Asia or the Pacific?

A Not immediately, except for the withdrawal of Japan from its occupied territories. What the war did was increase the discontent of people in colonial territories and accelerate their independence movements. By the end of the 1940s, India, Pakistan, Ceylon, Burma, Indonesia, the Philippines, and North Vietnam were independent, and other Southeast Asian countries soon followed.

TRUE OR FALSE?

The war made possible the creation of Israel.

PARTLY TRUE.

Zionists *had struggled to create a Jewish homeland in British-controlled Palestine since World War I. The arrival of hundreds of thousands of European Jews fleeing Nazi persecution made the Zionist movement strong enough to bring about Israeli independence in 1948.*

Stat: When the United States entered the war in late 1941, **1,801,101** men and women were in its military forces. When the war ended in 1945, **12,209,238** men and women were serving, and another **4 million** had left the service during the course of the war.

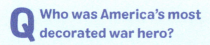

Q **Who was America's most decorated war hero?**

A **Audie Murphy (1925–1971) was the most decorated war hero. During his Army service in North Africa and Europe, he killed, wounded, or captured 240 enemy soldiers and won 28 medals. In 1955, his autobiography, *To Hell and Back*, was made into a movie in which he played himself.**

Q Was G.I. Bill a person?

A No. The "G.I. Bill" was a nickname for a federal law officially known as the Servicemen's Readjustment Act of 1944. The bill helped returning servicemembers readjust to civilian life. Its grants and low-interest loans enabled millions of veterans to attend college and buy homes, businesses, and farms.

Q What did the Marshall Plan do?

A Officially known as the European Recovery Program, the US plan provided nearly $13 billion (about $132 billion today) worth of aid to European countries between 1948 and 1952. Under secretary of state George C. Marshall's direction, it helped ensure the economic and political stability of Western Europe.

Q What made the Cold War cold?

A "Cold War" is the term for the intense post–World War II rivalry for world leadership between the US-led Western nations and the Soviet-led communist nations. It wasn't violent, but it wasn't exactly peaceful, either, as the rivalry intensified arms buildups. The Cold War ended with the breakup of the Soviet Union in 1991.

A In August 1941, even before the United States entered the war, British prime minister Winston Churchill and US president Franklin Roosevelt signed the Atlantic Charter, agreeing to help create a system to promote world peace. As the war expanded, nations joining the Allies signed the Declaration of the United Nations. In 1944, the alliance moved toward making itself permanent. A charter officially established the United Nations in San Francisco on October 24, 1945.

TRUE OR FALSE?

After the war, the German engineer most responsible for developing the V-2 rocket bombs that killed thousands of Allied civilians became a designer of US space rockets.

TRUE.

Rocket scientist Wernher von Braun became a US citizen after the war and later designed rockets used for the Apollo moon missions.

Did You Know?

Adolf Hitler's British-born nephew, William Hitler, served honorably in the US Navy during the war. Afterward, he changed his last name and spent the rest of his life in the United States.

Did You Know?

Truk Atoll, now known as Micronesia's Chuuk Lagoon, served as Japan's main South Pacific naval base during the war. In February 1944, US Navy planes sank 12 Japanese warships and 32 merchant ships in the lagoon. Thanks to the lagoon's clear water and huge collection of sunken ships and planes, scuba-diving tourism is now the atoll's main industry.

Did You Know?

Since 1939, more than 1,300 feature films have been made about World War II. Nine have won best-picture Oscars, including *Casablanca* (1943), *The Bridge on the River Kwai* (1957), and *Schindler's List* (1993).

GLOSSARY

Allies: A general term for countries fighting on the same side; when capitalized in reference to World War II, "Allies" refers specifically to the United States, the British Empire, the Soviet Union, and their allies

annexation: Adding part or all of a neighboring country's territory to one's own country

atomic bomb: A powerful nuclear weapon developed by the United States and used in warfare for the first and only time in history against Japan

Axis: An alliance among the Allies' three main enemies—Germany, Italy, and Japan

black markets: The illegal trade in goods not easily obtainable in legal markets

civilian: An ordinary person not in any military service

communism: A political and economic system promoted by the Soviet Union that favored complete government control over economic production and limited individual freedoms

concentration camps: Prison camps for civilians that Germany used to confine, mistreat, and ultimately kill millions of Jews and other peoples

convoy: A group of ships—military or civilian—sailing together for protection against enemy vessels, especially submarines

democracy: A political system in which leaders are elected by citizens and government protects individual freedoms

dictator: A ruler with unlimited power

fascism: A political system that favors strong government and extreme nationalism while opposing democracy and individual freedoms

fleet: Any group of naval warships under one commander

genocide: Deliberate efforts to destroy entire nations or ethnic groups

kamikaze: Japanese bomb planes whose pilots sacrificed their lives by piloting them all the way to their targets

Luftwaffe: The German air force

military auxiliary: An organization that supports a military branch but is not a full member of the military

nationalism: A strong belief in and support of the interests of one's own nation above those of other nations

Nazi: Abbreviated form of the German name of Hitler's National Socialist Party, used mainly by the party's opponents

neutral: Refusing to take sides in a war; Switzerland and Sweden were neutral in World War II

propaganda: Information—both accurate and inaccurate—put out by advocates of a cause or belief

radar: An electronic system for detecting and tracking distant objects, such as planes and ships

RAF: Great Britain's Royal Air Force

rationing: A government program for controlling the distribution of scarce goods, such as food and fuel, by limiting the amounts each person or family may purchase

Red Army: The official name of the Soviet Union's army

refugees: People forced to leave their own countries to escape oppression or other hardships

Resistance: Underground organizations in occupied countries, whose purpose is to resist and make things difficult for their enemies

sabotage: Deliberate destruction—usually secretive—of property or equipment by people working to make things more difficult for an enemy

sorties: Attacks made by a single military unit or aircraft; an attack made by five aircraft at once would be counted as five sorties

troops: A general term for small or large groups of soldiers

war crimes: Crimes that go beyond generally acceptable wartime behaviors; examples include genocide, abusing civilians, and mistreatment of prisoners

Zionists: Jewish people who believe that Palestine is "Zion," the original Jewish homeland to which they should return

RESOURCES

Want to learn more about World War II? Start here!

MUSEUMS

International Museum of World War II, Natick, Massachusetts

National Museum of World War II Aviation, Colorado Springs, Colorado

National Museum of the Pacific War, Fredericksburg, Texas

National WWII Museum, New Orleans, Louisiana

Pearl Harbor Aviation Museum, Honolulu, Hawaii

Rosie the Riveter WWII Home Front National Historic Park, Richmond, California

Wright Museum of World War II, Wolfeboro, New Hampshire

WEBSITES

History Channel (History.com/topics/world-war-ii)

National WWII Museum (NationalWW2Museum.org)

Smithsonian National Air and Space Museum (SI.edu/spotlight/wwii-aircraft)

US Department of Defense (Defense.gov/explore /features/story/article/2293108/significant -events-of-world-war-ii)

US National Archives (Archives.gov/research /military/ww2)

BOOKS

Adams, Simon. *DK Eyewitness Books: World War II.* New York: DK, 2014.

Catherwood, Christopher. *World War II: A Beginner's Guide.* London: Oneworld, 2014.

Halls, Kelly Milner. *Voices of Ordinary Heroes: A World War II Book for Kids.* Emeryville, CA: Rockridge Press, 2020.

Panchyk, Richard. *World War II for Kids: A History with 21 Activities.* Chicago: Chicago Review Press, 2002.

Roman, Carole P. *Spies, Code Breakers, and Secret Agents: A World War II Book for Kids.* Emeryville, CA: Rockridge Press, 2020.

ABOUT THE AUTHOR

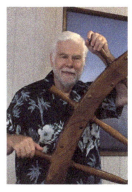 A former reference-book editor, **R. Kent Rasmussen** holds a PhD in history from the University of California, Los Angeles. In addition to the dozens of reference works he has edited, he has published more than 20 books of his own, including *World War I for Kids: A History with 21 Activities*, as well as five books on African history and 12 about Mark Twain.

CPSIA information can be obtained
at www.ICGtesting.com
Printed in the USA
JSHW012018310821
18310JS00002B/2